Book Title Copyright © 2020 by CW Piper.

This book is intended for information purposes only; it is not intended to be a substitute for professional medical advice.

Visit my website at *cwpiper.com*

Printed in the UK

Cover designed by CW Piper Designs

First Printing: March 2020
CW Publications

ISBN: 9798631936539

Imprint: Independently published

————————————————————

On Gut

Gut eats all day and lechers all the night;

So all his meat he tasteth over twice;

And, striving so to double his delight,

He makes himself a thoroughfare of vice.

Thus in his belly can he change a sin:

Lust it comes out, that gluttony went in.

BEN JONSON

CONTENTS

INTRODUCTION

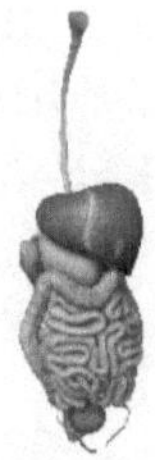

The gut is probably not one of the sexier parts of our body, and images of it can make us squirm a little, which possibly helps to explain why it has been largely ignored over time. However, it is a hugely important organ, and the intestines deserve our understanding and respect!

Our gut plays a key role in our overall health and well–being, and it is the source of many unexpected and fascinating facts concerning our human biology.

As long as we believe that we are healthy and the body is working properly, we don't give much thought to our digestive system and its main component, the digestive tract, the gut or guts. But if something does go wrong it will claim our attention fairly rapidly, and by then it may already be too late.

Our gut can influence much more than just our bathroom habits.

And what do we know about the gut? - for instance, of the two intestines we all have - you may know that the smaller small intestine is actually long, but did you know how long? If you unraveled it and spread it all the way out, it would cover a full tennis court (that's 2,800 square feet)! Such an enormous area is needed to efficiently absorb all of the nutrients in your diet, more on this later.

What is good for our guts? This lack of attention paid to our intestines, until very recently, has encouraged me to research the gut, and by writing this book, I will also educate myself in an area that I know little about before starting to explore. And hopefully documenting what I learn will demystify and educate you too.

As a brief introduction, and becoming more technical for a moment, and I promise to avoid doing this unless it is necessary, the *gastrointestinal tract* is an organ within us humans (and certain other animals), which takes in food, digests this food to extract and absorb energy and nutrients, and then expels the remaining waste as faeces or poop. So, our mouth, oesophagus, stomach and intestines all form part of the gastrointestinal tract.

The gut produces more than twenty different *hormones* to assist in this process, which in turn influence everything from our appetite to our mood swings. The gut even houses its very own 'brain' cells. These are known as the *enteric system*. It is, all in all, an exceptional piece of engineering, and we should show it due respect as a consequence.

Many facets of our modern life - such as high stress levels, too little sleep, eating processed and high-sugar foods, and the taking of antibiotics can all damage our gut microbiome. This in turn may affect other aspects of our health, such as the brain, heart, immune system, skin, weight, hormone levels, ability to absorb nutrients, and even the development of cancer.

One word of caution - tread carefully with all of the new advice that is being bombarded our way in recent years regarding probiotics, low-fat foods, antibiotics, and next – 'biome-friendly' foods, wherever possible, choose real food, ideally unprocessed, and where possible fermented foodstuffs.

Also, if you already suffer from any serious medical problems, such as coeliac disease, or show symptoms of such, I strongly recommend that you consult a medical professional before embarking on any major alterations to your diet.

A good start to any gut changing program is to keep a daily food diary to record your eating habits – you may be surprised at how easily this may help you to identify habits you were not even aware of, good or bad!

I have tried to keep this book interesting and easy to read, avoiding too much technical jargon and simplifying the language as much as possible.

I will begin by briefly explaining the human food digestion process to help understand the gut role in all of this.

Then I talk about the *microbiome*, how best to influence gut health, and what are the best foods to eat to help keep a healthy gut.

And I have devoted a whole chapter to discussing the phenomenon known as Leaky Gut Syndrome, as this is becoming a very topical theme nowadays, along with a section on gut disease.

I hope you find this information enlightening and useful!

1 – DIGESTION

It will help put the guts into context if I start with a brief introduction to the workings of the digestion system in humans. It is a surprisingly complex process, controlled by your other 'gut' brain.

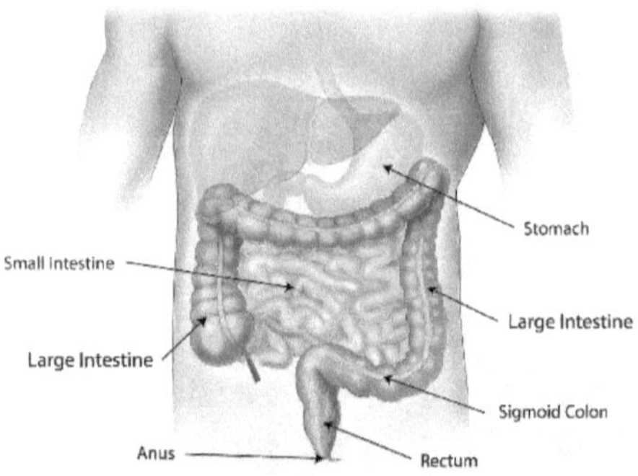

From our mouth then, food passes down through the pharynx to the (o)esophagus. This is a long muscular tube (25x3 cm) which connects through to the Stomach.

The stomach is a muscular sack, approximately equal to the size of 2 clenched fists, and sits just below your diaphragm, on the left side of your abdomen. It produces hydrochloric acid and enzymes which continue to break down the food just eaten.

Fluids pass through first, good if this is water or a beverage, bad if a sugar-laden drink (eg Cola). Like fluids, digestible carbs (eg bread, rice and potatoes) are rapidly absorbed. This may sound good, but the energy created will be immediate, and will pass quickly.

Protein-rich foods (eg eggs, wholegrain, meat and vegetables) are absorbed slowly, keeping you full for longer periods. Fibre from these foods will feed the good bacteria in your large intestine.

As an aside - the acid in your stomach would burn your skin, so why doesn't it burn your stomach? Well because a thick layer of mucus protects the stomach lining and keeps the acid on the inside, where it's churned with your food.

When gastric acid does sometimes leak up into the esophagus, which lacks this mucus layer, you will know that 'burning' feeling as heartburn.

Food then passes to the small intestine. This is another muscular tube, not that 'small' as mentioned (6x3 cm coiled) and made up of three parts – the *duodenum*, the *jejunum* and the *ileum*. It coils around like a hose, and the inner lining is covered in ridges allowing for maximum absorption.

It takes about 6 hours for food to pass through the stomach and small intestine, and in this time 90% of the nutrients have been absorbed.

Human digestive system

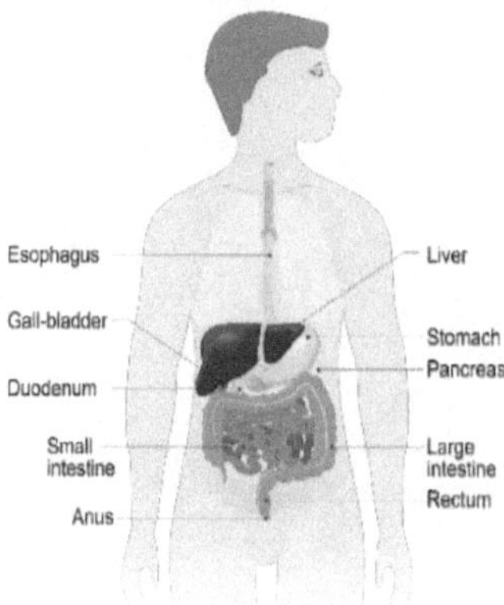

The large intestine comes next (1.5m x 8 cm), and this tube wraps around the loops of the small intestine. Its primary function is to absorb water. It contains approximately 2 kilos of good bacteria (gut flora), which will extract the last 10% of the nutrients.

Also made up of three parts – the *caecum*, the *colon*, and finally the *rectum*.

The time it takes for the remaining food to travel through these varies greatly from human to human, and it will depend on the food eaten (think of that spicy meal!). Interestingly, it tends to take longer in women than in men; a good average seems to be 33 hours and 45 hours respectively.

So, the rectum completes the digestive process.

2 – MICROBIOME

Microbiome is a term becoming more familiar in general usage these days, but what exactly is the microbiome?

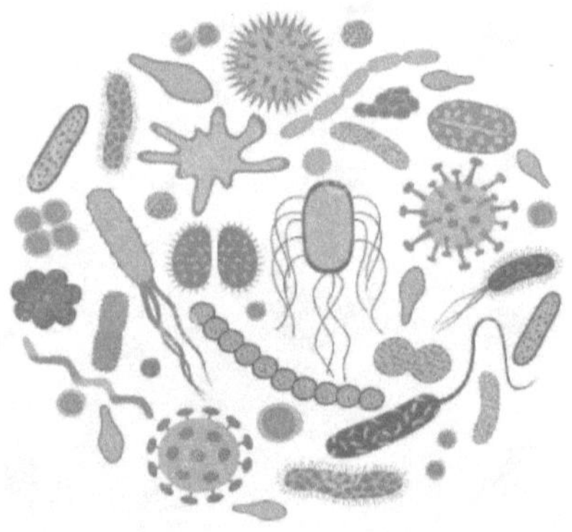

Microbiome is the term for a community of microbes, and our bodies are home to trillions of bacteria, viruses and fungi. These one or two kilos of microbes play a critical role in our overall health.

Microbes have existed for billions of years and they are everywhere, as well as within our bodies. For us they provide food, safeguard our health, and shape our bodies. Most of the microbes are found in a pocket of our large intestine (in the *cecum*), and they are referred to as the *gut microbiome*.

It is only in recent years or so that we have started to gain insights into the composition and function of these microbial communities – in fact with the help of development in DNA sequencing technologies.

There is still very little known about microbiomes across complex food chains - making it difficult to use this (DNA) technology to develop more sustainable food systems, and to develop innovative new products. While some bacteria are associated with disease, others are extremely important for our immune system, heart, weight and many other aspects of our overall health.

Although there are many different types of microbes, bacteria are the most studied. In fact, there are more bacterial cells in our body than human cells - roughly 40 trillion bacterial cells in our body and only 30 trillion human cells.

What's more, there are up to 1,000 species of bacteria in the microbiome, and each of them plays a different role in our body. Most of them are extremely important for your health, while others may cause disease.

Without the gut microbiome, it would be very difficult to survive. It begins to affect our body the moment we are born. Recent evidence suggests that babies may even come into contact with some microbes while inside the womb, rather than later when passing through the womb.

As we begin to grow, our gut microbiome begins to diversify, meaning it starts to develop many different types of microbial species. Higher microbiome <u>diversity</u> is considered good for our health. Naturally, the food we eat affects the diversity of our gut bacteria.

It starts to affect our body in a number of ways, including digesting breast milk (important for growth). Certain bacteria digest fibre, producing short–chain fatty acids, which are important for overall gut health. Fibre may also help prevent weight gain, diabetes, heart disease and the risk of cancer.

The gut microbiome also controls how our immune system works. By communicating with immune cells, it can control how our body responds to infection.

New research suggests that the gut microbiome may also affect the central nervous system, which controls our main brain function. This is a fascinating area of research and worth exploring.

The microbiome even helps us to decide which foods to have, and it also controls our hunger signals.

For a more in-depth understanding of the gut microbiome, there is more and more interesting information on available online, and you can explore in your own time, now that you have been introduced.

Bacteria

There are thousands of different types of bacteria in our microbiome, most of which benefit our health. However, having too many unhealthy microbes can lead to disease. An imbalance of healthy and unhealthy microbes is sometimes called *gut dysbiosis*, and it may contribute to weight gain.

Several well-known studies have shown that the gut microbiome will even differ between identical twins, thus demonstrating that our microbiome type is not necessarily genetic. The microbiome behaviour can be adapted however, as found in one study, when the microbiome from an obese twin was transferred to mice, they gained more weight than those that had received the microbiome of the lean twin, despite both groups eating the same diet.

As further studies show that microbiome dysbiosis may play a role in weight gain, adding probiotics to your diet is good for a healthy microbiome, and may help with weight loss. Other studies suggest that the effects of probiotics on weight loss are probably quite small. The jury is out.

The bloating, cramps and abdominal pain that people with IBS will experience may be due to gut dysbiosis. This is because the 'bad' microbes produce a lot of gas and other chemicals, which contribute to the symptoms of intestinal discomfort.

However, more healthy bacteria in the microbiome can improve gut health. They can help to seal gaps between intestinal cells and prevent *leaky gut* syndrome (see below).

Other bacteria within the gut microbiome can produce chemicals that may block arteries and lead to heart disease. Again, using probiotics may help lower cholesterol and the risk of heart disease.

The gut microbiome may also affect central brain health in a number of ways. Firstly, certain species of bacteria can help produce chemicals in the brain called neurotransmitters. For example, serotonin is an antidepressant neurotransmitter that's mostly made in the gut.

Secondly, the gut is physically connected to the brain through millions of nerves. Therefore, the gut microbiome may also affect brain health by helping control the messages that are sent to the brain through these nerves.

There are many ways to help improve your gut microbiome, including:

1. Variety – a diverse microbiome is an indicator of good gut health, so vary your diet. In particular, legumes, beans and fruit contain lots of fiber and can promote the growth of healthy *bifidobacteria*.

2. Reducing the amount of disease–causing species in the gut by eating fermented foods – such as yogurt, sauerkraut and kefir which all contain healthy bacteria, mainly *lactobacilli*.

3. Avoiding artificial sweeteners as evidence has shown that they can increase blood sugar levels by stimulating the

growth of unhealthy bacteria like *enterobacteriaceae* in the gut.

4. Introducing prebiotics – these are a type of fibre that stimulates the growth of healthy bacteria. Prebiotic-rich foods include artichokes, bananas, asparagus, oats and apples.

5. Breastfeeding is very important for the early development of the gut microbiome. Children who are breastfed for at least six months have more beneficial *bifidobacteria* than those who are bottle-fed.

6. Eating wholegrains – they contain lots of fibre and beneficial carbs like beta-glucan, which are digested by gut bacteria to benefit weight, cancer risk, diabetes and other disorders.

7. Eating less meat – yes, vegetarian food can help to reduce levels of disease-causing bacteria such as *E. coli*, as well as inflammation and cholesterol.

8. Eating food rich in polyphenols – these are plant compounds found in red wine (yes!), green tea, dark chocolate, olive oil and whole grains. They are broken down by the microbiome to stimulate healthy bacterial growth.

9. Adding probiotics - live bacteria that can help restore the gut to a healthy state after dysbiosis. They do this by "reseeding" it with healthy microbes. **You could consider probiotic supplements** if you find it difficult toad them easily to your diet regularly.

10. Resisting antibiotics – these treatments can kill many bad and good bacteria in the gut microbiome, also possibly contributing to weight gain and gradual antibiotic resistance. Thus, only take antibiotics when medically necessary.

In summary then, an imbalance of unhealthy and healthy microbes in the intestines may contribute to weight gain, high blood sugar, high cholesterol and other disorders.

The good news is that you can now discover more about your own microbiome by ordering a test online. The test will analyse all of the types of bacteria present in your sample and their relative proportions in your overall microbiome, and will provide information about the various functions of your gut bacteria, like the extent to which microbytes protect you against certain diseases and inflammation, as well as what vitamins they synthesise.

With your results, you will also get recommendations on how to improve and maintain the balance of your microbiome by adding specific foods to your diet.

Scientific research has established that bacteria in the microbiome are not simply 'good' or 'bad' species. Rather, how microbes participate in health or illness is dependent on their abundance in the overall community and how they relate to one another.

3 – HEALTHY GUT

So, what constitutes a healthy gut? Well there are a number of key factors to consider in improving overall gut health.

If you have symptoms such as cramping, bloating, abdominal pain, diarrhea, rashes, nausea, fatigue, or acid reflux, you may be suffering from a food intolerance. You can try eliminating common trigger foods to see if your symptoms improve.

If you succeed in identifying a food, or foods, that are contributing to these uncomfortable symptoms, you may see a positive change in your digestive health by changing your daily eating habits.

Food intolerance is the result of difficulty digesting certain foods (this is different than a food allergy, which is caused by an immune system reaction to certain foods).

It is thought that intolerances may be caused by the poor quality of bacteria in the gut as discussed earlier, which will lead to difficulty digesting the trigger foods and create unpleasant symptoms as per above.

Reducing Stress

Lowering stress levels is easier said than done obviously, but high levels of stress are hard on your whole body, including your gut. Some methods you can use to lower stress levels are meditation, exercise, walking, relaxing more and spending time with friends or family.

It may be no harm to decrease your caffeine intake (if you drink a lot of coffee).

Make a conscious effort to smile and laugh more, and consider taking up yoga or pilates, locally available courses are much more prevalent these days.

Another idea would be to get a pet, surprisingly rewarding if you have never tried this, and a great excuse to get more exercise in your day!

Sleeping

Not getting enough sleep, or a sufficient quality of sleep to allow recovery time after a busy day, can have serious impacts on your gut health, which can in turn contribute to more sleep issues – a vicious cycle.

Try to prioritise getting at least 7 or 8 hours of uninterrupted sleep every night. If you have young kids, grab those opportune moments for a quick nap during the day if possible, and ensure that you have a suitably comfortable and roomy bed to encourage sleep at night.

An unhealthy gut could contribute to sleep disturbances such as insomnia or poor sleep patterns, and therefore lead to chronic fatigue. The majority of the body's serotonin, a hormone that affects mood and sleep, is produced in the gut. So gut damage can impair your ability to sleep well. Some sleep disturbances have also been linked to risk for *fibromyalgia*.

If you are having problems sleeping, it may be a good idea to seek some medical advice in the short term.

Eating and Drinking

As well as having a good and well-balanced diet, try eating smaller portions and at more regular intervals. It is also very important to eat slowly - chew your food thoroughly to allow for steady and full digestion and absorption of all nutrients.

Reducing the amount of processed, high-sugar, and high-fat foods that you eat can contribute to better gut health. Additionally, eating plenty of plant-based foods and lean protein can positively impact your gut. A diet high in fibre has been shown to contribute tremendously to a healthy gut microbiome.

Proper eating habits will help you reduce or prevent digestive discomfort and maintain a healthy gut.

Drinking plenty of water during the day has been shown to have a beneficial effect on the mucosal *lining* of the intestines, as well as on the balance of good bacteria in the gut.

As well as water, hot drinks are important (not too much coffee remember) and make a conscious effort to limit, or eliminate altogether, the consumption of fizzy drinks during your day.

Supplements

Adding a prebiotic or probiotic supplement to your diet may be a great way to improve your gut health. Prebiotics provide 'food' meant to promote the growth of beneficial bacteria in the gut, while probiotics are live good bacteria. People with bacterial overgrowth, such as small intestinal bacterial overgrowth (SIBO, should not take probiotics.

Not all probiotic supplements are high quality or will actually provide benefit. It's best to consult your healthcare provider when choosing a probiotic or prebiotic supplement to ensure the best health benefit.

As long as everything in your digestion is working properly, you really won't have given too much thought to your digestive system and our guts. But it will claim your attention pretty rapidly when something does go awry.

Unhealthy Gut

There are many different ways in which an unhealthy gut might manifest itself. Here are some of the most common signs of poor gut health:

Stomach Upset – stomach disturbances such as gas, bloating, constipation, diarrhea, and heartburn can all be signs of an unhealthy gut. A balanced gut will have less difficulty processing food and eliminating waste.

Sugar Cravings – a diet high in processed foods and added sugars will decrease the number of good bacteria in your gut. This imbalance can cause increased sugar cravings, which can then damage your gut still further. High amounts of refined sugars, particularly high-fructose corn syrup, have been linked to the increased inflammation in the body. Inflammation can be the precursor to a number of diseases and even cancers.

Weight Swings – gaining or losing weight without making changes to your diet or exercise habits may be a sign of an unhealthy gut. An imbalanced gut can impair your body's ability to absorb nutrients, regulate blood sugar, and store fat. Weight loss may be caused by SIBO, while weight gain may be caused by insulin resistance or the urge to overeat due to decreased nutrient absorption.

Skin Irritations – skin conditions like eczema may be related to a damaged gut. Inflammation in the gut caused by a poor diet or food allergies may cause increased "leaking" of certain proteins out into the body, which can in turn irritate the skin and cause conditions such as eczema.

Auto-immune Conditions – medical researchers are continually finding new evidence of the impact the gut may have on the body's immune system. It is thought now that an unhealthy gut may increase systemic inflammation and alter the proper functioning of the immune system. This can lead to auto-immune diseases, where the body attacks itself rather than harmful invaders.

4 – GUT DIET

Diet and gut health are naturally very closely linked. Avoiding processed foods, high-fat foods, and foods high in refined sugars is an extremely important factor to maintaining a healthy microbiome, as these foods destroy good bacteria and promote growth of damaging bacteria.

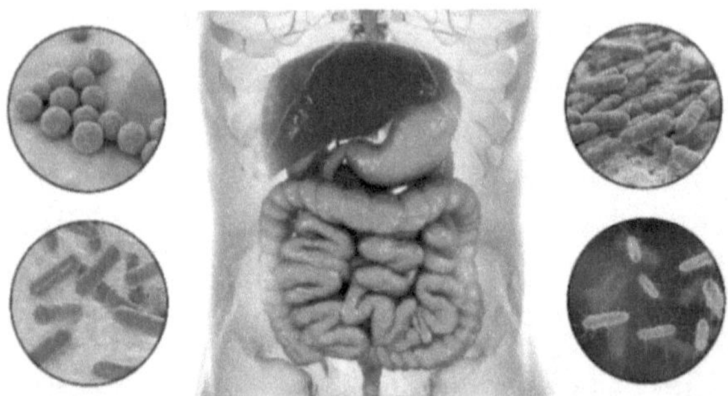

There are also a number of foods you can eat that will actively promote the growth of beneficial bacteria, contributing to your overall health. Introduced gradually into your diet, these foods include:

High-fibre

High-fibre foods such as legumes, beans, peas, oats, bananas, berries, asparagus, and leeks have always shown a positive impact on gut health in numerous studies.

Eating more fruit and vegetables will load more fibre of course and this is normally a good thing – so long as you have a healthy gut.

Some types of fibre are more important for your gut health than others.

It's easy to get caught up in counting calories and grams of added sugars, fats, proteins, and carbs when you're trying to eat well.

Scientists have long known that eating fibre is good for health. Decades ago, Irish physician (and fibre enthusiast) Denis Burkitt proclaimed, "*America is a constipated nation... if you pass small stools, you have to have large hospitals.*" And yet, years later, many of us are still ignoring our fibre intake.

American adults are only eating an average of 15 grams of fibre on any given day, despite the daily recommendations from the Academy of Nutrition and Dietetics being: 25 grams for women, or 21 grams if over 50 years old; 38 grams for men, or 30 grams if over 50.

Recently, however, fibre has popped up in headlines thanks to people like journalist Megyn Kelly and model Molly Sims, who have both credited their physiques on mainlining roughage. And more importantly, new research has been shedding more light on how fibre helps our bodies.

It has been linked to fending off disease and reducing the risk of a range of conditions, including type 2 diabetes, food allergies, and even knee arthritis.

Star-studded endorsements aside, it's not about eating a "high-fibre" diet as much as it's simply this: *eat more fibre.* Fibre does more than contributing to weight loss and reducing the risk of disease.

Losing out on those recommended fibre grams per day may significantly change the way your gut functions. It could even make a difference between weight loss or none, and longer life or not.

Prebiotics

Prebiotic fibres act as a compost to boost the growth of your good bacteria.

Inulin is the best known of these – found in the onion and garlic family – also dandelion, artichokes, asparagus and, yes, bananas,

Resistant starch – starch will 'resist' digestion in the small intestine, and then reach your colon largely intact!

Grain, seeds, unripe bananas, pasta, rice (cooled) - cooking, and cooling changes the structure of the starch in the pasta, rendering it more resistant to digestion! Reheating increases this effect even more.

Garlic and onions may have some anti-cancer and immune system-enhancing properties based on various studies, which are closely tied to some of the primary functions of the gut. Some of these benefits are anecdotal, although some research has been done.

Fermented foods such as kimchi, sauerkraut, yogurt, tempeh, miso, and kefir are great dietary sources of probiotics. While the quality of these foods may vary, their benefits on the gut microbiome are well studied.

Collagen-rich foods such as bone broth and salmon may be beneficial to overall health and gut health specifically. Many of these benefits are anecdotal conclusions and further research could be done. You could also try to boost your body's own collagen production through foods. Try adding a variety of foods, like mushrooms, good dairy, or certain meats.

The human gut is more complex than previously thought and has a huge impact on whole-body health. A healthy gut contributes to a strong immune system, heart health, brain health, improved mood, healthy sleep, and effective digestion, and it may help prevent some cancers and autoimmune diseases.

There are a number of lifestyle changes you can make to positively affect your gut health and your overall health as a result.

More About Fibre

Many studies have strongly linked high-fibre diets with longer and healthier lives. For instance, studies in the late 1980s found that long-living rural Japanese populations ate high-fibre diets, as opposed to urban dwellers with lower fibre intakes. But only recently have we gained a deeper understanding of why fibre is so vital to our well-being.

A 2017 study found that the importance of fibre is intimately tied with the importance of our gut microbes. A proper fibre diet literally feeds and makes these bacteria thrive. In turn, they increase in number and kind.

And as mentioned - the more microbes we have in our intestines (microbiome) - the thicker the mucus wall and the better the barrier between our body and our busy bacteria population. The mucus barrier lowers inflammation throughout the body, and the bacteria aid in digestion, creating a dual benefit.

A living example of the great connection between fibre, intestinal bacteria, and health are the Hazda, a Tanzanian tribe that are one of the last remaining hunter-gatherer communities in the world. They eat a spectacular 100 grams of fibre a day, all from food sources that are seasonally available. As a result, their gut biome is packed with diverse populations of bacteria, which ebb and flow with the changing of the seasons and the changes in their diet.

Your biome can change by the season, by the day, or even by the meal. And if you eat a large array of fresh fruits, grains, and vegetables, your gut health will reflect that. Eating low-fibre foods, or eating only a few types of fibre - such as the same fibre supplement every day - can in fact harm your intestinal biome and the health of your protective mucus wall.

However, eating too much fibre can also cause digestive distress, gas, and intestinal blockages. The good news is that it is quite difficult to get too much fibre, especially since most people don't get enough. Slowly ramping up your fibre intake can help you avoid some of the above problems. Not overdoing it will help you avoid the rest.

There are two types of fibre - soluble and insoluble fibre – and high-fibre enthusiasts are keen on both types. Each type has its own functions and benefits.

Fibre is naturally found in all fruits and vegetables and you can't really go wrong by adding a variety of (preferably) fresh fruit to your daily regime. In fact, one study found that simply eating an apple before every meal had significant health benefits, but the apple must not be chemically treated of course.

Always check your source is fresh, focus on in-season fruits and vegetables. Not only are they great for you, but they also often taste better and are less expensive than what's out of season.

Avoid processed food - refined foods that don't contain whole grains or whole wheat are also lower in fibre, such as white bread and regular pasta.

Juicing is also processed in a sense, since it removes the insoluble fibre from your food. The result is that you may remove and lose the fibre benefits -especially denying the important job of regulating digestion and keeping blood sugar from spiking.

Eating Out

Restaurants, especially fast-food joints, often skimp on fruits and vegetables because they are expensive. When looking at the menu, be sure to pick something rich in fruit, veggies, and beans or legumes that will help you meet your fibre goals for the day.

Next time you have a piece of pizza, maybe try to munch on a handful of snap peas on the side, or add some multigrain crackers if you're eating soup for lunch. Eating a high-fibre snack before your meal can also mean eating fewer calories altogether, because you'll feel more full.

And make it a habit to add beans, peas, and lentils to your regular diet.

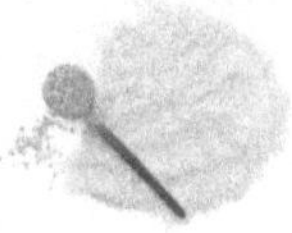

We often remember to eat our fruits and veggies, but legumes are a wonderful and delicious source of fibre. Try a recipe that puts legumes in the spotlight, like a three-bean vegetarian chili or a lentil salad.

Breakfast

Make a decision to start your day with some fibre. Most traditional breakfast foods, like eggs and bacon, actually lack fibre, so make some changes, and integrate fibre into the first meal of your day by eating oatmeal or a whole-grain cereal.

Or if you can't manage this try to remember to add a piece of fruit to your regular breakfast favourite. Eating yogurt for breakfast? Add sliced fruit and nuts.

Next time you visit the grocery store, pick up some bulgur, or pearl barley, or wheat berries, and start exploring. Other good high-fibre choices are quinoa (a seed) or whole-wheat couscous (a pasta).

Many people choose to add fibre supplements thinking this will be enough, and they will give you a small temporary boost, but the benefits of getting your fibre from whole foods are much greater. What's more, people taking fibre supplements might not be always pairing them with high-nutrient foods, and this causes rather than solves health issues.

At this point, there is enough science to strongly suggest something you've likely heard before: *eating a robust variety of minimally processed (fresh preferably) fruits and veggies along with other plant-based foods* is a great way to stay healthy and control your weight.

So, go ahead and reinforce the population and variety of bacteria in your gut, starting today!

Fructose Intolerance (IBS)

Studies show that a high percentage of people diagnosed with IBS have a fructose intolerance. This means their bodies have a reduced capacity to digest fructose (fruit sugar), as well as other sugars, starches and fibres.

To help people with fructose intolerance, a research team at Monash University in Melbourne developed a diet called the Low FODMAP Diet.

FODMAP is a rather un-tasty acronym (sorry), and it stands for – *fermentable oligo-, di- and mono- saccharides, and polyols* (!).

That is quite a mouthful (pardon the pun). To make it easier to understand, the main categories of foods that tend to aggravate IBS are:

- Fructose and fructans (in wheat and prebiotics)
- Lactose (a sugar in milk, and milk products)
- Galactans (in beans and lentils)
- Sugar and sugar alcohol (such as xylitol and sorbitol)

Even with fructose intolerance, a person can consume some amount of FODMAP foods. But when starting to follow a low FODMAP diet, it is best to become strict with your choices. Then, as you feel better, you can gradually add and experiment with different foods, to determine the amount your body can handle without causing IBS symptoms.

Another common cause condition associated with IBS is SIBO: Small Intestinal Bacterial Overgrowth. With SIBO, the bacteria that normally grow in small quantities in the small intestine begin to overgrow. Constipation, a common symptom of IBS, tends to make such overgrowth even more likely.

Food that is not digested well, emotional stress, and food poisoning also make you more susceptible to SIBO and IBS – and SIBO can lead to leaky gut (which we'll discuss next).

If you suspect you have SIBO, you can now do a SIBO breath test that measures the gases produced by the overgrowing bacteria. If you do have SIBO, it's a good idea to follow the low FODMAP diet as above... the diet can then be modified further to eliminate all starchy vegetables and grains (as they can feed the overgrowing bacteria) until your gut bacteria are back in balance.

5 – LEAKY GUT

Worth a chapter on its own, and termed 'intestinal permeability' in medical literature, leaky gut is when the cells that line the intestines become unhealthy, causing undigested food and other substances from within the intestines to 'leak' into the area located just outside the intestines.

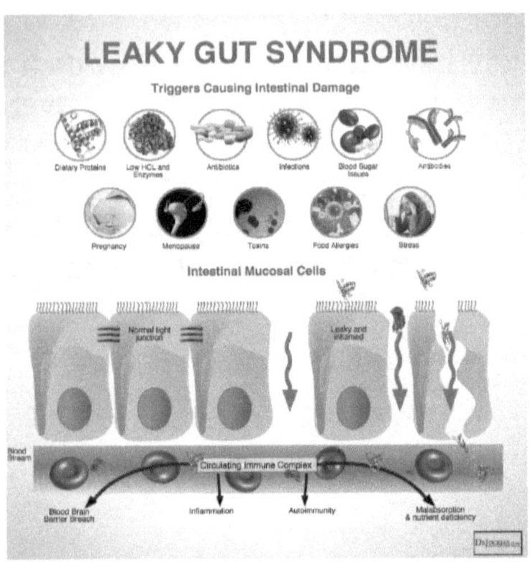

Leaky gut is caused by many factors including stress, pesticides, medication, gluten, and 'imbalanced' gut bacteria. If you already have leaky gut, coffee and alcohol can make it worse.

Nearly everyone with IBS has leaky gut too, but not everyone with leaky gut has IBS. Most of us have likely had some degree of leaky gut at a certain point in time, without realising it. You can think of the condition as a spectrum – from mild, to moderate, to severe. The more severe the condition, the more likely you'll feel unwell when you travel, and foods will upset your digestion.

Severe leaky gut can also predispose you to histamine (allergic) reactions, because the immune system gets triggered when it sees substances leaking outside the intestines into the blood stream.

Even without digestive symptoms or full-blown allergic reactions, leaky gut means your body is more likely to react to certain foods and to cause issues in other areas of your body (besides your digestion).

These reactions are called 'food sensitivities', and they are often triggered by the foods you may eat most often – such as gluten and dairy. When addressing leaky gut, it is still best to have a food sensitivity test done to find out which foods you need to avoid.

Lectins

Lectins are found in almost all of the foods we eat on a daily basis. These proteins bind to *carbohydratemolecules* (such as sugars) and have a variety of important functions in plants, animals and humans.

There are many types of lectins, and a few are toxic at high levels, according to the US Food and Drug Administration. 'High levels' is a key phrase here - because lectins bind to the carbohydrates that are available around them, the idea is that if there are a lot more lectins than carbs in the body, the leftover lectins may attach to the body's cell membranes and alter the cells' functions.

Most lectins are found in legumes. If you are cooking beans, grains and vegetables, the lectins are pretty much wiped out, and they are not going to affect your body. Probably the best known, and potentially most toxic type of lectin, is called *phytohaemagglutinin*, which is found at relatively high levels in raw beans. Eating as few as four raw kidney beans can cause vomiting and a host of other gastrointestinal symptoms, according to the FDA.

You might ask why you should take any chances with lectins. Why not just avoid anything containing these proteins? Well, there are several pieces of evidence hinting that we may need some lectins in our diet, and if you are lectin-free, you wouldn't want to eat pizza, for example. But never eat those raw beans, fully cook them to reduce their lectins.

The sugar-binding activity of these proteins means that consumed in ordinary amounts, lectins may even be necessary for normal digestion and absorption of foods. However, we have also evolved to eat foods that contain lectins. Lectins in modest concentrations in otherwise-healthy people may have advantages in reducing too-rapid nutrient absorption.

In other words, adopting a diet that eliminates lectins may alter nutrient absorption and result in severe nutrient fluxes.

There are also serious concerns about whether a lectin-free diet provides all the essential nutrients we need in modern life. Any time you are cutting out groups of foods, there is a possibility that you cut out things that are also good for you. Lectin, especially, is in so many fruits and vegetables that have disease-preventing characteristics.

Tomatoes, for example, have a strong antioxidant called lycopene that can actually have a number of positive effects on the cardiovascular system.

Moreover, studies looking at many thousands of people have documented the importance of plant-heavy diets for living a long, healthy life. And these diets would contain an abundance of lectin-containing foods.

When you are eating a plant-based diet, you are getting all of those anti-toxins and the variety of nutrients that are important for the gut microbiome to flourish and for you to live a long, healthy life.

A lot of lectin-containing foods, like grains and legumes, are also high in carbohydrates, so that people following a lectin-free diet are probably eating less of the foods high in carbs and high-glycemic foods.

A good first step, again, is to review your diet, making sure that you eliminate processed food - high-glycemic choices like white flour and pasta - and focus more on a variety of fruits and vegetables, lean meat and healthy fats.

As mentioned, and worth reiterating – to find out whether a particular ingredient in your diet is causing a reaction, dietitians will normally start by eliminating food types, and then reintroducing them one by one to check for a reaction to each item.

Lectins can come later as part of the process of elimination, and may not be an appropriate first step for most people. What is important to remember is that everyone is different and may respond in their own unique way to the various foods listed. What is one man's medicine can be another individual's poison. Try consuming these foods and pay attention to how your body responds to them. If you see unwanted symptoms, then stop eating that particular food!

6 – GUT CONTROL

"All disease begins in the gut" – was Hippocrates right when he made this bold declaration all those centuries ago?

Hippocrates, the father of modern medicine, was a wise man, and much of his wisdom, which is now over two centuries old, has stood the test of time.

To delve deeper, obviously not all disease begins in the gut. For example, this does not apply to genetic diseases. There is evidence these days, however, that many chronic metabolic diseases do, in fact, begin in the gut.

This has a lot to do with the different gut bacteria residing in our digestive tracts, as well as the integrity of the gut lining. According to numerous studies, unwanted bacterial products called endotoxins can sometimes "leak" through and enter the bloodstream.

When this happens, our immune system recognizes these foreign molecules and mounts an attack against them, resulting in a chronic inflammatory response.

This diet-induced inflammation may trigger insulin resistance (driving type 2 diabetes), leptin resistance (causing obesity), fatty liver disease, and has been strongly linked to many of the world's most serious diseases.

Keep in mind that this is an area of research that is rapidly developing. No clear answers have been discovered yet, and chances are that the science will look completely different in a few years.

Gut Inflammation

Just to make sure that we're all on the same page, I want to briefly explain what inflammation of the gut is, although it is actually a rather complicated topic.

It involves dozens of cell types and hundreds of different signaling molecules, all of which communicate in immensely complex ways. Put simply, inflammation is the response of the immune system to foreign invaders, toxins or cell injury.

The purpose of inflammation is to influence the function of immune cells, blood vessels and signaling molecules, to initiate an attack against foreign invaders or toxins, and begin repair of damaged structures.

We're all familiar with acute (short-term) inflammation. For example, if you get bitten by a bug, or hit your big toe on the doorstep, then you will become inflamed. The area will become red, hot and painful. This is inflammation at play. Inflammation is generally considered to be a good thing. Without it, pathogens like bacteria and viruses could easily take over our bodies and kill us.

However, there is another type of inflammation that may be harmful, because it is inappropriately deployed against the body's cells. This is a type of inflammation that is active all of the time, and may be present in your entire body. If is often called chronic inflammation, low grade or systemic inflammation.

For example, your blood vessels (like your coronary arteries) may be inflamed, as well as structures in your brain. It is now believed that chronic, systemic inflammation is one of the leading drivers of some of the world's most serious diseases. This includes obesity, heart disease, type 2 diabetes, metabolic syndrome, Alzheimer's disease, depression and numerous others.

However, it is not known exactly what causes the inflammation in the first place.

Study of the microbiome then could well be the most compelling frontier of health science. The digestive process breaks down food and beverage particles so that your body can absorb the nutrients it wants and excrete the rest. Trillions of organisms join in the effort.

The microbes also play a critical role in shaping your appetite, allergies, metabolism, and neurological function. And as we heard, scientists have found that gut bacteria produce neurotransmitters, such as serotonin, dopamine, and GABA, all of which play a key role in determining your mood.

Studies suggest that your gut microbiota may play a role in our risk of developing neuropsychiatric illnesses like schizophrenia, ADHD, obsessive-compulsive disorder, and chronic fatigue syndrome.

All in all, the bacteria living in our gut have a huge impact on the way we feel.

When it comes to the bacteria in your gut, every time you eat, you are feeding something. Unfortunately, the modern industrialised diet is all too often feeding the bad guys and, just as important, starving the good.

To put it simply, 'bad' bacteria tend to feed on sugar and unhealthy fats (yes, I'm talking about you, junk food!). And the single most important nutrient that good bacteria need to thrive inside you, as we discussed, is fibre.

When they have plenty of fibre, they can do their job – and your digestion, mental function, and even your mood reap the benefits.

It is clear then that fibre is critical to gut health. But sadly less than 5% of Americans, as an example, get the recommended 25 to 30 grams per day. It is estimated that our Paleolithic ancestors got an average of up to 100 grams per day.

Most of us are literally starving the good bacteria that would, if we only gave them the chance, be digesting our food and making the brain-boosting chemicals we need to thrive.

We know that junk food, lack of fibre, glyphosate, antibiotics, and other toxins can compromise the bacteria upon which our digestion and brain health depend.

There is a lot we can do to nurture a healthy microbiome and to support a flourishing collection of beneficial bacteria in our digestive tract.

A diverse population of health-promoting flora protects our gut from the less helpful strains.

Feed the good ones

The word probiotic comes from the Greek meaning 'support of life'.

Probiotics are the so-called 'good' micro-organisms inside our gastrointestinal tract. They aid in digestion and keep our tummy happy. Like all living things, probiotics must be fed in order to remain active and vibrant.

Prebiotics are the food that probiotics need to thrive. They're a type of plant fibre that humans can't digest, and that take up residence inside our large intestine. The more of these prebiotics we feed to our probiotics, the more efficiently they'll do good work inside us.

The simplest way to think of it is this: if you want to nurture good bacteria, eat lots of fibre. Whole plant foods – especially fruits, vegetables, legumes, and whole grains – have the most fibre.

People interested in fostering a health-promoting array of gut micro-organisms should consider shifting from a diet heavily based on meats, carbohydrates, and processed foods to one that focuses on plants.

If our probiotic bacteria were in charge of the menu, they'd want abundant sources of prebiotic fibres like inulin and oligofructose, as well as pectin, beta-glucans, glucomannan, cellulose, lignin, and *fructooligosaccharides* (FOS). If you don't know how to pronounce these names, don't worry. Luckily, you don't need a degree in biochemistry to eat good food.

Some top superfoods that provide an abundance of the best microbe-fueling nutrients include: gum arabic (sap from the acacia tree, often sold as 'acacia fibre' , chicory root, baobab fruit, dandelion greens, garlic, leeks, and onion, asparagus, wheat bran, bananas, apples, barley and oats, flaxseed, cocoa, and seaweed.

The 2 main ways to consume probiotics are in fermented foods or in dietary supplements. Probiotics have been found to be helpful in treating IBS, diarrhea, colitis, acne, and eczema. But they don't always work. Hence, a lot of people are taking probiotic supplements that are pretty much just a waste of money in my opinion.

The challenge is that the vast majority of probiotic bacteria are active and effective in the lower portions of the gastrointestinal (GI) tract, but to get there, they must survive the corrosive and highly acidic environment of your stomach.

Researchers attempted to settle this question with a study reported in the journal Beneficial Microbes a few years back.

The team built a fake digestive tract with a fake stomach and intestines, but complete with real saliva and digestive enzymes, acid, bile, and other digestive fluids. They put probiotic capsules into this stomach 'empty' and with a variety of foods, and then tested how many survived the trip.

What did they find out? Probiotic bacteria had the highest rates of survival when provided within 30 minutes before or simultaneously with a meal or beverage that contained some fat.

This makes sense. Consuming probiotics with food provides a buffering system for the bacteria, helping to ensure safe passage through the digestive tract. But consuming them after a large meal could slow everybody down, making bacteria more likely to die in the corrosive stomach environment before reaching their intended new home in the lower intestine. So right before, or with, a meal that includes some fat seems the best way to go.

Fermenting

Fermentation helps to preserve food and creates beneficial enzymes, B vitamins, and numerous strains of probiotics.

Natural fermentation has been shown to preserve nutrients and to break some foods down to a more digestible form.

The most studied is kimchi, a traditional Korean food made from fermenting salted cabbage with a variety of vegetables and spices (sometimes salted shrimp or anchovy is included, as well).

In addition to, or perhaps because of, its probiotic properties, studies have shown that kimchi can help fight cancer, obesity, effects of aging, and constipation while contributing to your immune system, skin health, and brain health.

Other popular fermented foods include sauerkraut, yogurt (which can be made from cow, soy, coconut, or almond milk), kefir, miso, natto (made by boiling and fermenting soybeans with bacteria), beet kvass (a fermented beet drink), vinegar, and kombucha.

Some fermented foods are used in condiments, while others make a tasty snack or topping. But remember not to cook them if you want to preserve the probiotics.

Keep in mind that some probiotic kefirs and yogurts come loaded with added sugar. Even if there are beneficial bacteria in these probiotics, the sugar will feed the 'bad' bacteria already in your gut. Always check labels for sugar content.

If you want to do your own fermentation, I recommend finding a good book or website to guide you. One book to consider is 'Fermented Vegetables' by Christopher and Kirsten Shockey.

Some people using homemade fermented foods are experiencing great benefits after moving to a whole-food, plant-powered diet that features an abundance of fermented foods, such as kimchi, fermented vegetables, tempeh, homemade almond milk yogurt, and miso.

7 – SPICE FOR THE GUT

I love spices, and am pleased to report that spices have been used throughout history as digestive stimulants.

In recent times, studies have shown that many spices stimulate the liver, resulting in it secreting bile that has a higher percentage of bile acids. Bile acids are important for fat digestion, as well as absorption, so making sure you have enough of them is important.

Spices have also been found to stimulate the activities of pancreatic lipase, protease, and amylase. These enzymes help support a more efficient digestive system.

Some spices also help improve food transit time in the gastrointestinal tract. A sluggish gastrointestinal tract allows time for more water to be absorbed out of the digested food; this can result in painful constipation. Additionally, the longer digested food is allowed to sit in your system before it is eliminated, the more prone it is to be preyed upon by unhealthy bacteria.

Ginger

Ginger contains phenolic compounds which are known to relieve gastrointestinal irritations. It stimulates saliva and bile production. Animal studies have also demonstrated that ginger prominently enhanced intestinal lipase activity, which is an enzyme used in digestion.

Ginger reduces intestinal contractions by relaxing the intestinal muscles and allowing digested food to pass more easily. In fact, it reduces cramping of the stomach and bowels and may even help with menstrual cramping.

Ginger is good for reducing gas and bloating and is famous for addressing other gastrointestinal distress, such as nausea due to morning sickness and chemotherapy. Unlike Dramamine, ginger can stop your nausea without making you sleepy.

The *zingiberaceae* botanical family, which ginger is a part of, also includes turmeric and cardamom, which are both incredibly healthy spices themselves.

My favourite dishes to add ginger to are my warming soups.

Many people drink ginger tea in the morning to wake up their sluggish digestion. I also sometimes add it to water, tea, or even hot water with lemon when I am traveling to settle things down after too much hotel food, or simply for a refreshing, cleansing drink.

Note that ginger does have a blood-thinning action, so it should be used with caution by those taking blood-thinning medications. And you may want to avoid consuming ginger for two weeks prior to surgery and another week following surgery. Check with your doctor.

Coriander Seeds/Cilantro

Coriander seeds, which yield cilantro, have been used for thousands of years to help with digestion. Both coriander seeds and cilantro are healthy, but the seeds contain more health benefits for digestion.

Coriander has carminative properties, which means it helps with gas. It is also known to have antispasmodic and stomachic properties. It calms intestinal spasms that can lead to diarrhea so it may be helpful to some people having irritable bowel syndrome. Coriander can also help settle indigestion.

As an added benefit, cilantro is packed with phytochemicals, which are super antioxidants. It is also used to lower blood sugar and is being studied in animals for its potential cholesterol-lowering benefits.

Cilantro has also been researched as a heavy metal detoxifier. In rats, it has shown to suppress lead accumulation.

Coriander is sold in whole seeds and in powdered form. I always buy the seeds, as the oils dissipate very quickly once they've been ground, usually within a few months.

Use coriander as a delicious rub in stews, pickled dishes, and marinades. You can also add it to soups and smoothies.

Fresh cilantro is wonderful in hot and spicy dishes because of its cooling effect. Just chop up a little cilantro and throw it in whatever dish you are cooking. It encourages the production of supportive digestive enzymes that break down your food.

Cardamom

Cardamom is part of the ginger family, so no wonder it's helpful for your digestion.

It has been used in Chinese and Ayurvedic medicine for centuries but is also backed by science as having actions that help relieve bloating and gas (aka carminative properties). It also has antispasmodic properties, as it can slow the rate of stomach muscle cramping.

Cardamom also stimulates the appetite along with easing gas, nausea, indigestion, and cramping. It helps to kill off any food-borne bacteria in the digestive tract, thus helping to protect against food poisoning and gastric distress.

Cardamom pods contain a compound called limonene, which is usually found in citrus peels. It is known to dissolve cholesterol-containing gallstones, as well as relieve heartburn and gastroesophageal reflux (GERD).

Cardamom also has antioxidant benefits, as well as being a good source of minerals, such as iron, manganese, calcium, and magnesium.

Cardamom works well as a diuretic and can reduce bloating, water retention, swelling, and edema. It is often used in sweet and savoury dishes. And it can be prepared as a delicious, warming tea by placing four cardamom pods in two cups of water and simmer for 30 minutes. Sweeten with stevia, if desired.

Cardamom pods can be chewed on to relieve tooth and gum pain, as well as prevent infection.

Fennel Seeds

Fennel stimulates the production of gastric juices and is another great spice having carminative properties. It is often used as an after-dinner digestive aid. It also has antispasmodic properties.

Fennel seeds are a very rich source of dietary fiber as well. It consists of metabolically inert insoluble fiber, so it increases the bulk of the food you eat as it goes through your digestive system. This eases constipation problems. Its fiber helps protect your colon.

Fennel also contains a variety of antioxidants, such as quercetin, which is thought to offer protection from aging and diseases, including cancer.

A good trick (thanks to my friend and peer, Dr. Alan Christianson) to reduce bloating and gas, is to heat fennel seeds on low in a skillet with some sea salt.

Let them get slightly brown, and then store them in a tightly closed container. You can add a few pinches of these slightly cooked seeds to any of your dishes. It really works!

Other Spices that Help

Turmeric – this Indian spice aids digestion while soothing your digestive tract. It has been found to help relieve heartburn, reduce stomach pain (due to its anti-inflammatory and antibacterial compounds), reduce flatulence, and more.

Cumin – cumin is another great spice for digestion and is great for heartburn.

Lemon Balm – one of my digestive spice favorites is lemon balm!

Garlic - has so much to contribute to the gut immunity.

Fenugreek - fenugreek acts as a natural digestive and helps flush out toxins from the body.

Cinnamon Bark - warming cinnamon bark is a mild but useful remedy for sluggish digestion. The German Commission E recommends it for loss of appetite, dyspeptic complaints, bloating, and flatulence.

There are other great spices for improving digestion. Just go to a reputable herb and spice shop online and do a little of your own research. You'll find that a lot of the Italian spices are also good for digestive support.

And go a little wild - find some new tastes that also will help your tummy and lead to a healthy gut.

A recent study has found that our modern lifestyle, diet and overuse of antibiotics are causing an increasing disruption of the gut microbes that are the basis of our immune system.

What is going on in your intestines or gut is an essential part of your health. In fact, remember your gut and your immune system are very closely linked, with 70 to 80% of your immune tissue situated in your digestive tract.

Because our intestines are inside our bodies, most people don't realise that it forms a protective barrier between our bloodstream and the external world. What's inside your gut is actually "outside" your body.

The gut has to deal with the pathogens in everything you ingest and therefore needs to have an effective immune system in place to ward off attacks and prevent illness.

The gastrointestinal immune cells are known as "Peyer's patches" and protect the mucous membranes of the small intestines against infection by releasing white blood cells (T-cells and B-cells).

Boosting the action of the immune cells are certain strains of gut flora that prevent pathogens from being absorbed. This is why it is so important to have colonies of 'good' bacteria in the gut. In fact, without the right balance of gut flora your body cannot maintain good health.

Breastfeeding is very important because it colonises the gut of the newborn baby with good bacteria from the mother which is associated with a decreased risk of allergies and other problems of the immune system.

Apart from serious disorders like autoimmune diseases, a strong immune system reduces the number of colds and flu and other antigenic conditions that plague the human race.

When the integrity of the gut is compromised, it can lead to that 'leaky gut', where the body is no longer protected against 'invaders' like undigested food, gluten and bacteria which have passed through the "holes" in the gut lining.

Coeliac disease is a lifelong condition caused by an immune reaction to gluten, resulting in inflammation of the gut lining an auto-immune disease rather than an allergy or an intolerance.

Gluten is found in wheat, barley and rye. It is relatively common (1 in a 100), but many people never know they have it.

So then, processed and junk food, and too many antibiotics, will destroy many of the good gut bacteria. This has led to the proliferation among the modern generations of food allergies, intolerance to certain types of food, and even obesity.

CONCLUSION

Healthy microbiome, healthy gut, healthy body.

Topical nowadays – as well as protecting ourselves from any virus on the outside, we can also build up our defences from the inside by strengthening our immune system. The immune system is complex and highly responsive to the world around us, so it's not surprising that many factors affect its function.

We can control the health of the trillions of microbes living in our gut, our microbiome, which plays such an essential role in the body's immune response to infection and in maintaining overall health. As well as mounting a response to infectious pathogens like the coronavirus, a healthy gut microbiome also helps to prevent potentially dangerous immune over-reactions that damage the lungs and other vital organs.

These excessive immune responses can cause respiratory failure and death. This is also why we should talk about "supporting" rather than "boosting" the immune system, as an overactive immune response can be as risky as an underactive one.

A diverse microbiome is a healthy microbiome, containing many different species that each play their part in immunity and health. Microbiome diversity declines as you get older, which may help to explain some of the age-related changes we see in immune responses, so it's even more necessary to maintain a healthy microbiome throughout life.

As we have discovered then, the best way to increase microbiome diversity is by eating a wide range of plant-based foods, which are high in fibre, and limiting ultra-processed foods including junk food. Following a Mediterranean diet has also been shown to improve gut microbiome diversity and reduce inflammation: eating plenty of fruit, vegetables, nuts, seeds and whole grains; healthy fats like high-quality extra virgin olive oil; and lean meat or fish.

Avoid too much alcohol, salt, sweets and sugary drinks, and artificial sweeteners or other additives. If you are concerned about getting hold of fresh produce while self-isolating or quarantined – frozen fruit, berries and vegetables are just as healthy as their fresh counterparts, and will last much longer than the recently recommended two-week isolation period. Canned fruit, beans and pulses are another long-lasting option.

You can also support your microbiome by regularly eating natural yoghurt and artisan cheeses, which contain live microbes (probiotics). Another source of natural probiotics are bacteria and yeast-rich drinks like kefir (fermented milk) or kombucha (fermented tea). Fermented vegetable-based foods, such as Korean kimchi (and German sauerkraut) are another good option.

So, finally, my summary advice, in bullet form:

- ❖ Eat a wide variety of foods

- ❖ Avoid drinking too much, moderation is best

- ❖ Stop smoking

- ❖ Limit your use of non-essential medicines

- ❖ Get a good night's sleep

- ❖ Avoid stress if you can

- ❖ Get enough daily exercise.

Useful References:

http://www.sciencemag.org/news/2015/08/gut-microbes-linked-eye-disease

https://www.elsevier.com/books/the-gut-brain-axis/hyland/978-0-12-802304-4

https://en.wikipedia.org/wiki/Human_digestive_system

https://study.com/academy/lesson/small-intestine-nutrient-absorption-and-role-in-digestions.html

https://www.elsevier.com/books/the-gut-brain-axis/hyland/978-0-12-802304-4